Aloje

ALL ABOUT
THE MENOPAUSE
AND ITS
TREATMENT
WITHOUT DRUGS

ALL ABOUT
THE MENOPAUSE
AND ITS
TREATMENT
WITHOUT DRUGS

By David Potterton ND, MRN, MNIMH
Consultant Medical Herbalist and
Registered Naturopath

foulsham

LONDON • NEW YORK • TORONTO • SYDNEY

foulsham
The Publishing House
Bennetts Close, Cippenham, Berkshire, SL1 5AP

ISBN 0-572-02154-2

Phototypeset in Great Britain by Typesetting Solutions, Slough, Berks
Printed in Great Britain by St. Edmundsbury Press, Bury St Edmunds.

Contents

Going Through The Menopause Naturally

Plants contain everything that the human body requires to function properly – they provide both food and medicine.

Those used for medicinal purposes contain vitamins, minerals and trace elements as well as a range of other constituents, including natural antibiotic compounds, hormones and hormone-like substances.

Some plants contain components that act on the body rather like oestrogen or progesterone, although the plant may not contain either of these hormones. In the case of oestrogen, for example, these substances are said to be oestrogenic.

Herbalists, using their powers of observation over the years, have identified many of the plants that act in this way.

In more recent times these observations have been confirmed by chemical analyses.

However, herbalists are not so much interested in the individual chemical components of their remedies as they are in how the total ingredients of a single whole plant, or a number of plants, work together to restore health and wellbeing.

Using isolated chemicals as drugs is not the province of herbalists. Their skill lies in making accurate clinical observations and selecting the correct remedies for a particular individual after taking a full case history.

As a professional group, herbalists in Britain have by far the most *clinical* experience of any in the world. This is because in many other countries where herbal remedies are valued they are frequently prescribed by physicians – the physicians are also the herbalists.

In Britain and the United States, however, physicians and pharmacists turned their backs not only on herbal medicine, but also on the importance of foods and diet in disease, scorning them in favour of the chemical approach.

Now that this approach is increasingly being shown to be flawed, there has been a revival of traditional methods and remedies and a growing respect for the professionalism of qualified herbal practitioners.

Herbalists have shown that plants contain not only hormones, but ingredients from which the body can itself produce hormones. Indeed, some of the most effective herbs for menopausal and other hormonal conditions contain not a trace of a hormone.

This book explains the menopause in simple language and discusses how the distressing symptoms associated with it can be treated by natural methods, provided that the condition has been properly diagnosed.

Many of the remedies mentioned are available from herbalists or health food shops, while others may be obtained only after a consultation with a medical herbalist or naturopath.

Complete success with natural methods may entail a degree of self-motivation as some change in lifestyle is usually involved.

It is strongly recommended, however, that should any doubts about treatment arise it is advisable to seek the personal advice and encouragement of a qualified practitioner. *This book is not intended as a replacement for proper medical diagnosis and care, and should not be regarded as such.*

There are certain dangers with the self-diagnosis of the menopause as this is the time of life when other serious illnesses can occur, the symptoms of which may resemble those of the menopause.

Note: Because it is recognised that there are contra-indications and that individuals may react differently to herbal remedies, the author and publishers emphasise that they cannot be held liable for any adverse effects caused by self-treatment with any of the remedies mentioned in this book. Self-treatment must be undertaken according to the individual's own judgement.

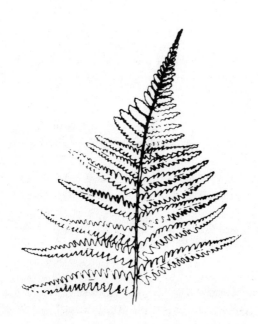

Words of Caution

Herbal medicines are generally safe, but they are not without contraindications. Therefore, the following general rules should be observed:

1 Never take any herbal medication during pregnancy without advice from a qualified practitioner.

2 Do not treat babies and young children, or the very elderly, without obtaining professional advice as dosages are much more critical.

3 Do not take herbal medicines without advice if you are also taking medicines from your own doctor, as the two may interact.

4 Do not self treat if you are suffering from a liver condition, heart problem, or other serious disease.

5 Always use herbs and herbal products from reputable herbal medicine suppliers, but preferably from a medical herbalist.

6 Do not gather medicinal herbs from the wild. Do not use other than culinary herbs from your garden.

7 Self-medication should be undertaken only for short periods of time and for simple conditions. Do not self-treat undiagnosed conditions.

Chapter 1

The Menopause Syndrome

In medical circles the menopause is now regarded as a syndrome. It is not just the cessation of periods that marks this phase of life, but a whole set of conditions, ranging from hot flushes to osteoporosis.

The advent of the syndrome coincides neatly with the introduction of hormone replacement therapy, which is seen by some doctors, and of course pharmaceutical companies, as the treatment of choice for all these conditions.

The menopause – or more accurately the climacteric – is seen to comprise symptoms which precede the menopause, such as breast tenderness, those which mainly accompany the cessation of periods, such as hot flushes and disturbed emotional states, those associated with degenerative changes in the skin and reproductive organs, such as skin dryness and loss of vaginal elasticity, and those described as metabolic, notably brittle bone disease or osteoporosis.

All these conditions are considered to be hormone deficiency states, requiring the prescription of hormone replacement therapy – either synthetic oestrogen alone, or a combination of oestrogen and progesterone.

While all these conditions are associated with hormonal decline, not everyone is agreed that synthetic hormones are the treatment of choice. Why is it, for example, that a great number of women sail through the menopause without any difficulty whatsoever? The answer, according to recent research, may be in the diet that they follow.

Despite intense campaigning in medical journals to persuade doctors to give menopausal women hormone replacement therapy, and despite the fact that some doctors will do so at the drop of a hat, most physicians and their patients are not entirely happy with this form of treatment and some are highly suspicious.

It seems that although nine out of ten women with menopausal symptoms seek their doctor's advice, one in five receive no treatment and only three out of 100 are referred to a hospital menopausal clinic.

Of those who do receive treatment from their GPs, one in three is put on to tranquillisers and antidepressants or similar drugs. The rest receive HRT, but only on a short-term basis.

In London, for example, less than 10 per cent of post-menopausal women who are given HRT stay on it for more than three years, while in Glasgow only about three in every 100 women on HRT stay on it for this length of time.

This is remarkable when one considers the near-monopoly that GPs enjoy in dealing with their patients' ills and how marvellous HRT is said to be by its proponents.

Obviously there are good reasons for this lack of enthusiasm, not least the fear that HRT may possibly be associated with cancer.

But there is also the problem that women on HRT still have a monthly, albeit artificial, period. Only about one in four women think that this is a price worth paying out to obtain relief from menopausal symptoms, while four out of five doctors say that it is a major drawback in pre-scribing it.

What should be remembered is that the menopause is not a disease – it is a normal phase of life. With natural treatment it is possible to pass through this phase without symptoms, or with only minimal symptoms, as women have done for centuries.

Of course, it must be accepted that symptoms can be very severe in some women and, consequently, more difficult to treat, but this is not a good reason for putting the whole of the World's middle-aged women on to HRT, especially when the vast majority are never given the opportunity to try natural methods first.

Herbal medicine and naturopathic treatments have much to offer and, logically, should be the first treatment of choice.

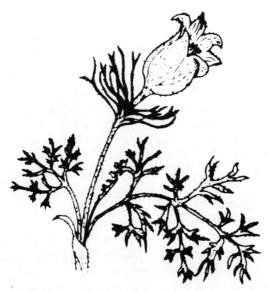

Pulsatilla

Chapter 2

It's Your Age!

Why do women experience the menopause at different ages? The answer seems to be that like the onset of menstrual periods the age is subject to a number of factors, including the woman's general health, her nutritional status, and even the society she lives in.

In Britain the median age – the age at which most women go through the menopause – is between 50 and 52.

Sometimes the menopause occurs abruptly, the period normal one month and absent the next; more commonly the periods become lighter and occur less frequently; while some women experience heavier and irregular bleeding, a condition known as menopausal menorrhagia.

When this occurs it is always essential to investigate the cause of the bleeding to rule out the possibility of a serious disease, such as cancer of the uterus. Women who regularly attend for smear tests should have little to fear.

Among the symptoms that may accompany the menopause are hot flushes and dizzy spells, depression, nausea (rather like that of pregnancy), insomnia and headaches and a reduced interest in sexual activity.

The woman may also complain of dry skin, vaginal prolapse, and vaginal inflammation.

As hormone levels of oestrogen and progesterone decline, the woman who has not kept herself fit and healthy is more likely to experience prolapse of the bladder or uterus.

Although the onset of the menopause is still regarded by some women as the end of their sexual lives, this is a myth. Many women find that without the worry of the monthly period they experience a far more satisfying sexual relationship.

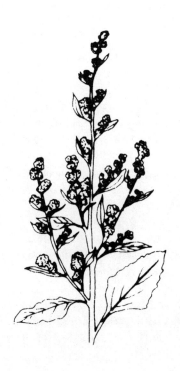

Chapter 3

Hormones and the Heart

Most doctors believe that oestrogen protects women from coronary heart disease. The argument for this is that the incidence of heart attacks in menstruating women is much lower than it is for men.

But after the menopause, when oestrogen production has virtually ceased, the heart attack rate in women increases dramatically and becomes much the same as for men.

One of the benefits of hormone replacement therapy, it is argued, is that it gives women protection against heart disease. This benefit, with other postulated benefits, is said to outweigh any adverse risk, such as cancer.

Although there is a possibility that this may be true, there really is a lack of real evidence to confirm this.

Why, if oestrogen therapy is so protective, is it contra-indicated for women who have a history of heart disease, or who suffer, have suffered, or are at risk of circulatory and thrombotic diseases, such as thrombophlebitis, stroke, high cholesterol, high blood pressure and varicose veins?

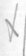

Why is it necessary to check the blood pressure regularly during hormone treatment and, if it is found to be raised, withdraw the treatment?

It seems that all the women who are at risk of heart disease are not, or should not be, receiving hormone replacement therapy.

That leaves on HRT only women who are considered not to have any risk factors.

Would it not be surprising then if the statistics for hormone replacement therapy were affected by this to show that fewer women on HRT suffer heart disease?

I seem to recall that when the contraceptive pill was introduced there was said to be an association between heart disease and oestrogen, which is why the combined oral contraceptive was supposed to be an advance.

Yet a history of thrombosis or angina or other heart or circulatory disorders are still contraindications for the combined Pill.

In the light of all this it doesn't seem to make sense to say that hormone replacement therapy is protective of the heart, but this is exactly what the "experts" are saying. However, I have never met any woman who has been put on to HRT specifically in order to protect her heart.

Obviously there are better ways of protecting one's heart than taking HRT – like taking more exercise, following a healthy diet, not smoking, dealing with stress problems and, if necessary, reducing body weight.

What's more, none of these natural alternatives has any risk factor attached to it.

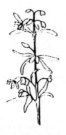

Rosemary

Chapter 4

Does HRT Cause Cancer?

The major worry for middle-aged women who are prescribed hormone replacement therapy by their doctors is: "Does it cause cancer?".

There have been so many conflicting reports over the years about a possible link between oestrogen and cancer, and between cancer and HRT, that it is no surprise that doctors themselves are confused about the possible risks.

There seem to be two groups of doctors – one is enthusiastically promoting HRT while the other is reluctant to prescribe it.

I will try in this chapter to present some of the arguments and factors involved in the controversy.

We need to go back to the mid-1890s for our first clue to a link between cancer and hormones.

In those days radical mastectomy was the treatment of choice for breast cancer, but some specialists noted that in cases where it was impossible to perform a mastectomy, removal of the ovaries sometimes improved the course of the disease.

By removing the ovaries, oestrogen production is dramatically reduced, which implies that there is some connection between the severity of breast cancer and oestrogen.

In young menstruating women removal of the ovaries,

whether or not they have breast cancer, results in an artificially induced menopause, complete with menopausal symptoms.

Although mastectomy is still used today, there is in many cases a chemical option – a drug which acts against oestrogen. This is used to try and slow down the course of the disease.

The drug is also given to older women with breast cancer who are well past the menopause, and in whom one would suppose oestrogen production had virtually ceased.

The side effects experienced with anti-oestrogen therapy are, not surprisingly, similar to menopausal symptoms and include hot flushes.

A further consideration is that breast cancer tends to be a much more aggressive disease in young menstruating women who are producing oestrogen than in those who are through the menopause and who have low levels of the hormone.

Among other evidence for a link between cancer and oestrogen is that oestrogen is chemically similar to known cancer-producing agents, and that cancer in laboratory-bred animals seems to be much more common if oestrogen is administered to them.

It might seem strange then that some specialists are now claiming that oestrogen administration is protective against cancer in general, although there is some doubt about cancer of the uterus.

The guidelines on hormone replacement therapy for the menopause, for example, recommend that if the woman has not undergone hysterectomy (and, therefore still retains her uterus), she should not be prescribed oestrogen on its own as this *might* lead to uterine cancer.

Current practice is to combine the oestrogen with progesterone. But if a woman at the menopause has already undergone a hysterectomy the guidelines say that she may be prescribed oestrogen alone.

So does oestrogen cause cancer, or does it not? The perplexing factor is that if it did one would expect cancer to be more common in younger women than in older women. But the reverse is the case – both cancer of the uterus and breast cancer are much more common in older women who have low levels of oestrogen.

In pregnancy, when oestrogen levels are at their highest, breast cancer is not unknown, but it is rare.

So it seems that oestrogen itself may not cause cancer. Indeed, it would be difficult for a naturopath to accept that a hormone that is naturally produced by the body could cause cancer. It just does not make sense.

But that does not answer the question at the start of this chapter – Does hormone replacement therapy – as distinct from hormones produced naturally by the body – cause cancer? If it doesn't why are anti-oestrogens prescribed as a treatment in breast cancer?

One theory is that oestrogen does not cause cancer, but that when a tumour develops in a susceptible person the hormone seems to accelerate its growth.

This is an interesting theory and may very well be true, but there are other factors to take into consideration.

For example, there is a postulated link between the over-consumption of fat and cancer. It has been suggested for many years that people who are overweight may be at an increased risk of deveoping breast cancer.

Conversely, all forms of cancer are much lower in strict vegetarians, who tend to be under-average for weight.

Strict vegetarians would also, of course, not be consuming animal products which have synthetic hormones injected into them.

Another consideration is that the hormones prescribed

for the menopause, or for that matter, any other condition, are not natural. Many of them are artificially produced in the laboratory. Some are derived from animals.

Dosage may also be important. It is practically impossible to supply the body with the exact dose it needs at any given moment. One is either going to have too much or not enough – and probably on a long-term basis.

When the contraceptive pill was first introduced under the banner of "scientific medicine", for example, women were taking in a single dose more oestrogen than they take now in a whole month's supply. What effect that has had on cancer statistics we may never know.

In the light of current knowledge and taking into account the prescribing guidelines there is no doubt that there is a real cancer risk to some women from oestrogen replacement therapy, but that this is apparently reduced, or prevented, when progesterone is added to the formulation.

There is a current argument among some specialists that hormone replacement therapy is contraindicated for the menopause in women with breast cancer, yet it is all right to give it to women at risk of breast cancer, or to women that have had breast cancer in the past.

This argument, put forward not only by some gynaecologists, but cancer specialists as well, is that "the benefit in reducing menopausal symptoms outweighs the risks".

Among the risks that are being referred to, apart from breast cancer, are osteoporosis and heart disease.

The fact is, however, that despite dozens of clinical trials on the possibility of an association between oestrogen therapy and breast cancer there is still no agreement among "the experts" as to who might and who might not actually be at risk.

Overall, however, it does appear that the longer a woman uses hormone replacement therapy the greater the risk of cancer developing. This is estimated to reach a one-in-three chance after 15 years of use.

In women with a family history of breast cancer it is three out of four.

We must conclude that the picture is far from clear. It would indeed be an understatement to say that further research needs to be done, not only to evaluate all the various oestrogen and combined hormone preparations being prescribed, but also the dosages used, particularly as they are being taken by millions of women all over the world.

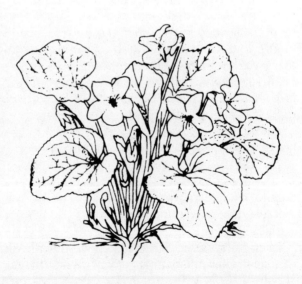

Chapter 5

Hot Flushes

The hot flush is the most frequently reported menopausal symptom, probably because it is the one that most women can obviously link to the change in their hormonal status.

Changes in mood that often accompany fluctuations in hormonal function may be more subtle and may not so easily be associated with the menopause.

A hot flush is usually described as a sudden sensation of heat that flows through the body – but mainly the chest, neck and head – like a wave and is often accompanied by the appearance on the skin of red patches. There is sweating, sometimes severe, which as it subsides, leaves the woman with an unpleasant chilly feeling.

Flushes are particularly disturbing at night and the perspiration produced may be so drenching as to require the bedclothes to be changed.

The number of flushes ranges from one or two a day to every half hour, while the individual flush may last just a few seconds or up to half an hour. In some women the flush may last for an hour or more.

Stress, anxiety and excitement, all tend to aggravate the flushing.

In medical terms hot flushes are said to result from vasomotor instability. This merely means that the nerves supplying the tiny muscles in the walls of the blood vessels which regulate the calibre or size of the vessel – whether it is dilated or constricted – are in some way interfered with, but precisely how is not quite clear.

One line of thinking, however, is that there is a disturbance in the balance between the hypothalamus, a centre in the brain concerned with the release of hormones, and the autonomic nervous system, which governs bodily functions that take place automatically, like the heart rate. It is as if they suffer a kind of withdrawal symptom as circulating oestrogen levels go into a decline.

Obviously in dealing with hot flushes one needs to take account of the stresses and strains of modern living and the anxiety levels it produces as well as combatting the flushes by dietary methods and herbal medicines as described in this book.

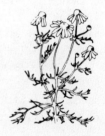

Wild Chamomile

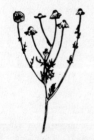

Common Chamomile

Chapter 6

Herbs and the Menopause

Professional medical herbalists use a number of herbs in the treatment of hormonal conditions, including the menopause.

Many of these herbs are sources of natural hormones, including oestrogen and progesterone. But which herbs are prescribed will depend entirely on the menopausal symptoms being suffered by the individual woman.

Quite often, nervine tonics which help to allay anxiety and generally settle the system down, may be prescribed for hot flushes. Sometimes it is necessary to include a circulatory tonic in the prescription to deal with symptoms like palpitations. Medicines which tone up the pelvic organs – that is both the musculature and the blood circulation – are frequently used to regulate menstrual upsets in the pre-menopausal years.

Some of these herbs are dealt with individually on the following pages. Chapter 20 (p.63) lists herbs which have various uses and may be helpful in an individual case.

Herbs have a long history of use for hormonal conditions and have been well documented down the ages. Modern herbal medicine utilises not only remedies which were popular in ancient civilisations, and found to be still of value today, but also those which are used by people who have stayed with their traditional approaches to medicine in various parts of the world, but particularly China, India and South America.

Chapter 7

The Herbal Hormone Regulator

An extract from a dark purple berry, produced by a shrub growing in Mediterranean countries, has been used by herbalists for years for treating conditions associated with an approaching menopause.

The medicine is regarded as a hormone regulator, although the berry does not iteself appear to contain any hormones.

The leaf-losing shrub is known as the Chaste Tree because the Greek physicians believed that administering the medicine would maintain chastity in young maidens. It was thought that it would quell the fires of passion, thus preventing them from succumbing too early to sexual overtures.

In some towns flowers from the shrub are still thrown to the ground in front of young men or women entering a monastery or convent.

The Romans considered the tree to be sacred and used the herb in fertility rites to Ceres, their goddess of agriculture.

Many of the ancient physicians, including Hippocrates, Dioscorides and Galen, mention its use as a remedy "for female complaints".

In recent times, its reputation as a remedy for hormonal complaints has been re-investigated, mainly by researchers in Germany.

They found that it was, indeed, a useful remedy not only for hormonal imbalances in pre-menopausal women, but also for menstrual irregularities and premenstrual tension in younger women.

One of their earliest findings was that it helps to produce milk in breast-feeding mothers.

The remedy today is known among herbalists as *Vitex*, which is derived from the Latin name for the shrub. It is one of the most frequently prescribed herbs, mainly because it covers a wide spectrum of symptoms, ranging from cyclical migraine to swollen ankles. The symptoms, however, all have one thing in common – they are due to hormonal imbalance.

Research spanning 45 years or more has revealed that the extract made from the berries, which look like small currants or peppercorns, influences the circulating levels of oestrogen and progesterone by acting on the system which controls the release of these hormones into the blood.

It also boosts the level of prolactin – the milk-producing hormone – in nursing mothers; stimulates production of luteinising hormone (LH); and inhibits release of follicle stimulating hormone (FSH).

It is FSH which stimulates the ovaries to produce oestrogen and LH which stimulates ovulation and the production of progesterone.

The way that Vitex treats hormonal imbalance is easier to understand if you think of an electric convector heater with a thermostat. As the room warms up the heater switches itself off and the room begins to cool. As it cools, the heater switches on again. If there was an imbalance the room would become too hot or too cold.

Hormones operate in much the same way. Oestrogen increases in the blood to a certain level when an automatic process inhibits its production and stimulates progesterone instead. Then, when progesterone reaches a certain level this is "switched off" in favour of oestrogen again, the whole process taking about 28 days.

If the system gets out of balance as it may do prior to the menopause, due to shocks or upsets, or, as I believe, to the ingestion of synthetic hormones from animal food sources, it is not surprising that a woman will complain that her hormones are "playing up".

The best way to take Vitex is in the form of a tincture available on private prescription from a medical herbalist. It is very simple to take – one dose a day is usually sufficient.

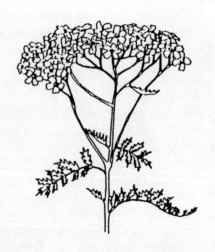

Yarrow

Chapter 8

Making Mothers Merry

A treatise on herbal medicine for the menopause would not be complete without the inclusion of Motherwort, which as its name suggests has been observed down the centuries to be of particular value as a pick-me-up tonic for mothers. It is frequently prescribed to ease menopausal symptoms such as heart irregularity, nausea, hair loss and depression.

The famous 17th Century English herbalist, Nicholas Culpeper, summed up its usefulness when he said: "It makes mothers joyful", and, "There is no better herb than this to take melancholy vapours from the heart".

The Latin name for Motherwort, *Leonurus cardiaca* gives perhaps a better indication of how this herb might act, cardiaca being a reference to the herb's affinity for the heart.

It is generally used by modern herbalists as a simple relaxing heart tonic, in cases, for example, where a woman complains of palpitations. But it appears to act on the heart via the nervous system, rather than directly on the heart muscle. So that where anxiety or nervousness affects the smooth functioning of the heart, Motherwort will, by a reflex action, settle things down by allaying the anxiety.

This ability to settle the patient down explains its popular use in earlier days for the restlessness which so often accompanies fevers and, today, as a valuable remedy where a general quietening down of the system is called for.

Motherwort is also indicated for a number of other heart and circulatory conditions. Dizziness due to low blood pressure, for example, is helped because of the tonic or strengthening effect of the herb on the heart.

Interestingly, low blood pressure is seldom regarded by English physicians as a disease, whereas in Europe, particularly in Germany, doctors have a wide range of remedies to choose from for this condition. It seems to have been noticed that patients who suffer from low moods frequently have a lower than normal blood pressure.

Patients with over-active thyroids which affect heart rhythm are also given Motherwort in combination with other remedies.

In younger women, Motherwort is used as a remedy for pre-menstrual tension, as a uterine tonic and to improve the menstrual flow.

And, although it has been used during pregnancy for certain conditions, its ability to "bring on the menses" tends to make it unsuitable for women who are liable to miscarry during pregnanacy.

The plant, which grows to about a metre in height, belongs to the same family as mint, but does not have that pleasant minty taste. Indeed, it is rather bitter.

Although it is a native European plant, I have never seen Motherwort growing wild. But it will grow quite happily in an English garden and is quite an attractive perennial.

For medicinal purposes, the tincture prescribed by herbalists is the recommended way of taking it. Do not expect immediate results – it can take a few weeks to do its work.

Chapter 9

Secrets of the Squaws

A herb long used by the American Indians to treat various menstrual complaints has, in recent times, been found to contain active principles resembling oestrogen.

The American Indians simply called it Squaw Root, but it is now known to herbalists across the United States and Europe as Black Cohosh.

Although a member of the buttercup family, the plant bears little resemblance to the small plant that we know here.

It is a tall, hardy, herbaceous perennial, bearing long graceful spikes of white flowers in late summer. Like the buttercup, however, it produces a tangle of creeping roots and it is these that are used medicinally.

Herbalists, who refer to the plant by its botanical name, *Cimicifuga racemosa,* make fluid extracts and tinctures from the roots, which they use in prescriptions for oestrogen-deficiency conditions.

The plant does have a number of other medicinal uses, however, including the treatment of blood pressure.

DEPRESSION

As a treatment during the menopause, Squaw Root, or Black Cohosh, has been found to be useful in relieving the depression which so often occurs at this time of life.

Indeed, as a herbal remedy it is generally categorised as a nervine tonic rather than as a hormonal agent.

Unfortunately, it may not act immediately and may, therefore, have to be taken for some time. In this case, it is best taken under the direction of a medical herbalist.

The American herbalists traditionally used Black Cohosh for a number of conditions affecting the ovaries and uterus, including painful periods and to relieve pain in childbirth.

However, as it is also considered to be a useful remedy for bringing on the menstrual flow when the periods have been suppressed – it would be contraindicated in pregnancy in women who are apt to miscarry.

In any event dosage is restricted as overdoses may produce nausea and vomiting.

SQUAW VINE

Another useful American Indian remedy is Squaw Vine, which is generally used as a uterine tonic. Known to herbalists as *Mitchella repens*, it seems to improve circulation and muscular function of the uterus. It is helpful when the menstrual cycle becomes disrupted, as it so often does in the pre-menopausal years, and the menstrual flow is either too little, too much, or causes pain.

Squaw Vine was a traditional American Indian remedy for easing childbirth, which it does by strengthening the pelvic organs. Although I do not have information regarding the hormonal content of this herb, the action is undoubtedly hormonal.

Given to men it reduces the involuntary discharge of sperm.

The herb is taken as a decoction, or in tincture form available from herbalists.

SQUAW WEED

A traditional remedy for menstrual irregularities, but still widely used, Squaw Weed *(Senecio aureus)* is usually combined with other agents in the treatment of menopausal upsets.

Like Squaw Vine, it helps when the menstrual flow is too scanty, or too profuse. Although not considered to be a powerful emmenagogue, it is contraindicated in pregnancy. *Correct dosage is important* – large doses may irritate the liver – and, therefore, it is recommended that this herb be taken only on prescription from a qualified medical herbalist. The herb is also prepared homoeopathically, but again is available only on prescription from homoeopathic clinics.

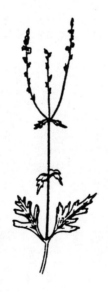

Vervain

Chapter 10

No Sweats

There are many herbs that are recommended for their ability to increase sweating. These are useful, in fevers for example, to help lower the temperature by bringing the body's internal heat to the surface.

Conversely, common Sage has the ability to reduce sweating and, indeed, was frequently prescribed in the days when tuberculosis was rampant to help relieve the night sweats associated with the disease.

In recent years herbal research has uncovered the fact that Sage contains hormonal substances which are similar to oestrogen and which act on the body in a similar way.

The presence of these oestrogenic substances, plus its ability to relieve sweats, has popularised Sage as a remedy that can be used at the menopause, particularly where hot flushes are a problem.

Herbalists, being extremely observant, reported the hormonal and gynaecological effects of Sage centuries before the discovery of hormones.

Culpeper, in the 17th century, for example, noted that a decoction of the leaves and branches of the plant "brings down women's courses" – in other words it promotes the menstrual flow. He also noted that it "expels the dead child". In Ancient Egypt Sage was used to improve women's fertility.

Modern herbalists advise that Sage, despite it being a common kitchen herb, should be avoided as a medicinal remedy during pregnancy, because of its action on the womb. However, it has been used by mothers for centuries to stop breast milk being produced when the baby has tired of the breast and is being weaned onto solid foods. It is likely that Sage interacts with prolactin, the hormone mainly involved in generating breast milk.

Sage has other uses in the gynaecological field, including the treatment of painful periods, and vaginal or uterine discharge. It is strongly antiseptic, and the infusion used as a vaginal douche is often recommended.

Although it has been a popular culinary and medicinal herb for centuries in Britain, it is not a native plant. It was imported originally from the Mediterranean countries where it grows wild.

There are many varieties of Sage, the one used by herbalists being known as *Salvia officinalis*. This is important as the infusion of some varieties induces sweating rather than inhibiting it.

It is a shrubby plant growing to about 60 centimetres high with woody stems, grey-green wrinkled leaves, which are sometimes reddish-purple, and blue or purple flowers.

As a bonus, Sage is also good for those with poor digestion, which is why it has become a culinary herb. It is a useful remedy for dyspepsia and flatulence.

The infusion being antiseptic makes a simple but effective gargle in sore throat and laryngitis.

The tincture is usually prescribed by herbalists for internal use during the menopause in combination with other remedies, depending on the requirements of the individual case.

Some care is required with Sage as overdosing can give rise to toxic symptoms.

Chapter 11

Unwind With Nervines

The exact hormonal basis of the emotional disturbances accompanying the menopause is unclear, yet we only have to think of the post-natal depression that affects many younger women, to realise that hormones and feelings are intricately bound up.

Many women are confused because they cannot tell whether their hormones are dictating their feelings and moods, or whether their feelings are upsetting their hormonal system. They do not know whether what they feel is reality, or whether their suffering is due to a bodily disturbance.

The same is true of vitamin and mineral deficiences – iron deficiency being the best known example. Although there are often physical symptoms such as cramps and weakness, there is often only an irritability or depression that is difficult to interpret.

Herbal medicines have an important role to play in helping to sort out these feelings. Not only do they contain minerals and vitamins, but they also contain substances which help body and mind to relax. Herbalists classify such remedies as nervine tonics.

One of the more important is Lady's Slipper, also known as nerve root and American valerian.

It is a delicate wild orchid which at present is in very short supply and, therefore, highly expensive.

However, it is a most effective remedy for nervous and emotional disorders associated with the menopause. It is a natural relaxant, working directly on the autonomic nervous system.

Herbalists, who know it by its botanical name, *Cypripedium pubescens,* prescribe it, usually in tincture form in combination with other remedies, for a wide range of nervous states – from acute hysteria to insomnia and for painful conditions affecting the nerves, such as neuralgia and nervous headache. Like Motherwort it is indicated for nervous palpitations and rapid heart rate.

Combined with Black Willow Bark it dampens down *excessive* sexual desire, although a lack of desire is more often the complaint during the menopause.

It is hoped that this plant will be allowed to flourish once again in the future, so that its valuable properties can be available to more people.

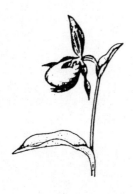

Lady's Slipper

Chapter 12

Menstrual Medicine

Although mainly prescribed as a kidney remedy, Shepherd's Purse has a reputation as an effective medicine where the menstrual periods are disturbed.

Its importance lies in its ability to control bleeding. It is prescribed not only for menstrual upsets, but also for haemorrhages from various parts of the body, including urinary tract, lungs, nose and bowels. It is understood, of course, that a proper diagnosis must be made in these cases.

The main drawback with Shepherd's Purse is its taste, which cannot be described as pleasant, but the usual method of overcoming this if taken in tincture form is to add it to fruit juice or a favourite herb tea.

The plant, known to herbalists as *Capsella bursa-pastoris,* will control excessively heavy periods or, as Culpeper said – "it will stop the terms in women". It is indicated in the pre-menopausal years for bleeding fibroids.

These benign uterine growths are dependent on oestrogen for their survival, which is why hormone replacement therapy is contraindicated in women that suffer from them. Once the menopause has arrived, however, fibroids tend to shrivel up of their own accord because of the oestrogen deficiency.

Shepherd's Purse gives relief when menstrual periods

are painful and is also used for benign uterine haemorrhages not associated with menstruation, a condition known as metrorrhagia.

For domestic use an infusion is made of the dried herb – one ounce to 20 fluid ounces of boiling water – and taken in doses of 2 fl oz.

As the plant contains tyramine it may not agree with people who suffer from migrainous headaches.

WHITE DEAD NETTLE

The White Dead Nettle *(Lamium album)* has some similarities with Shepherd's Purse and may be combined with it. For example, it has been used for uterine bleeding and it also contains tyramine. It was once a popular treatment for simple vaginal discharges, the infusion being used as a douche or taken internally.

Culpeper was particularly irritated that the physicians in his day called the plant Archangel "to put a gloss on their practice" and to conceal from their patients that they were just being given a common herb that they could so easily find for themselves.

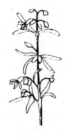

Rosemary

Chapter 13

Soothes and Slims

Fennel has had a long history in herbal medicine, and has been used by all age groups, from babies to the elderly.

Its properties were well known in ancient times when it was valued as a sight restorer and as a slimming remedy. The Greeks called it marathron which means to grow thin.

One of its earliest uses was undoubtedly as a settler of upset stomachs. It was an ingredient of compound liquorice powder, which was given as a laxative, the Fennel helping to prevent griping. Today, fennel water is still used to ease colicky pains in babies.

The ever-observant professional herbalists, however, discovered that it had a number of hormonal actions. It was noticed, for example, that breast-feeding mothers who partook of Fennel invariably produced an abundance of milk and, not only that, the babies seemed to enjoy their feeds more. Culpeper recommended that the leaves or seeds be boiled in barley water and drunk for this purpose. He also reported that medicines made from the seeds help to bring on the menstrual period.

The essential oil, which is extracted from the plant, but mainly the seeds, has similar properties, but like most essential oils should be taken only under the supervision of a practitioner due to its extreme potency.

It is now known that Fennel has oestrogenic properties

which has verified the plant's use as a remedy during the menopause. Herbalists prescribe tinctures made from the seeds.

The various uses of this particular herb demonstrate the impotence of so-called scientific research which causes panic by identifying a substance in the plant, feeding it to animals in massive quantities, and then warning that it could be dangerous to humans.

Fennel is a remedy that has been given to babies for centuries to soothe and calm their digestive systems, it is a kitchen herb that is regularly eaten with fish, while at the other end of the spectrum, the essential oil can be toxic. It is not a list of substances in a plant that is important so much as how they are used medicinally.

Fennel is one of the more pleasant-tasting remedies and, although its oestrogenic action may be variable, it has found service down the centuries for women who require a simple treatment for menopausal discomfort.

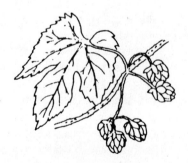

Hops

Chapter 14

And So To Bed . . .

Traditional Hop pillows are well known for helping sufferers of insomnia to get a good night's sleep. The aroma given off by Hops is certainly relaxing and sleep inducing.

It is reputed that King George the Third, when he suffered flare ups of a mental illness, was given a Hop pillow to help him to sleep.

Herbalists tend not to prescribe Hop pillows, as such, but make strong fluid extracts and tinctures from the plant, which they prescribe, often with other remedies, to help people get a good night's rest.

Hops are an ideal complementary remedy for women who are plagued by hot flushes which disturb their sleep, for not only do Hops relax the central nervous system, they also contain considerable amounts of oestrogenic hormones, especially when freshly picked.

This means that herbalists need to extract the active principles of this herb at exactly the right time if it is to be effective.

Hops are used extensively by the brewing industry, and the plant, a climbing vine, is cultivated in most parts of the world. Hop pickers, who are exposed to the plant for a whole season, often complain of symptoms which are similar to those of oestrogen excess, such as headache and tender breasts.

In herbal dispensaries the plant is known by its botanical name *Humulus lupulus*. The oestrogenic substances are extracted from the strobiles, or female flowers of the plant.

The hormonal attributes of the plant also explain its successful use in treating painful menstrual periods.

Traditionally, Hops have been classified as a nervine tonic and sedative, and were used to treat hysterical states, but they are also useful as an indigestion remedy and as a liver and gall bladder tonic. Correct dosage is important.

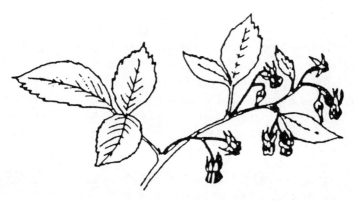

Raspberry

Chapter 15

True and False

Two American herbs, both used by herbalists in the treatment of menstrual and hormonal conditions, are commonly known as Unicorn Root, which can be confusing.

Although both members of the lily family, they are different plants. To differentiate between them, one is called the True Unicorn and the other the False Unicorn.

However, like many herbs they are also known by a number of other common names. This is why medical herbalists always use the botanical, or Latin names. There should then be no danger of the wrong herb being ordered or prescribed.

The True Unicorn, known to herbalists as *Aletris farinosa,* grows both in North Africa and in the United States, preferring a wet, swampy environment such as the coastal districts north of Florida. It produces white, bell-shaped flowers on stems about three feet tall.

The medicinal properties are found in the root, but herein lies another lesson very common in herbal medicine – the properties of the fresh root are not the same as the dried.

Herbal students are taught not only which parts of a plant are the right ones to use, but also what preparation the plant needs to undergo before it is suitable to use as a medicine.

If used fresh, True Unicorn root will induce vomiting. It also acts as a cathartic, and may cause abdominal pain as well as a feeling of being drunk.

When the root is properly dried, however, it becomes a valuable menopausal tonic – some would say one of the best available. It has a number of indications, but is particularly suitable for the menstrual upsets and debility that occur at this time.

It is one of the few herbs that helps with prolapse of the pelvic organs and with the back pain that may accompany this condition.

In younger women it is used to normalise menstrual periods whether they are heavy, absent or painful. It is also a remedy that helps prevent miscarriage.

Smallish doses of this herb, usually in tincture form, are generally prescribed with other remedies, depending on the individual condition and, therefore, it is best taken under the supervision of a qualified practitioner.

False Unicorn Root is also known as Helonias. Even botanically it has more than one name, but is most commonly known as either *Chamaelirium luteum* or *Helonias dioica*. I favour the latter.

Like the True Unicorn, the False also prefers to grow in damp ground. The medicinal properties of the dried root are also similar. It is an emetic and should be used only in small doses.

A valuable uterine and vaginal tonic, it is indicated for menopausal problems such as prolapse, but also for heavy periods and anaemia.

Like True Unicorn it can be given to younger women to help prevent a miscarriage. Once again it is recommended that this medicine be taken only under the supervision of a qualified herbalist.

Chapter 16

Homoeopathic Remedies

Homoeopathic medicines are extremely useful in treating certain aspects of the menopause. Many people are under the impression that herbal medicine and homoeopathy are one and the same thing. However, nothing could be further from the truth.

While herbal remedies are produced from extracts from plants, the source of homoeopathic medicines may include not only plants but a wide range of vegetable, animal and inorganic materials.

Homoeopathic remedies are also given in dilution rather like a vaccine. The principle is that a small amount of the chosen medicine will switch off the symptoms that would be produced by giving the raw material in an excessive amount.

Thus, if a particular substance taken to excess causes flushing, a dilution of the substance made into a homoeopathic medicine should, if it is given correctly, act like a vaccine and reduce the flushes.

Before the advent of a vaccination for smallpox, it was known that if a person sniffed the skin scales collected from a smallpox victim, it would increase their resistance against the disease.

It must be said, however, that some homoeopathic practitioners stretch this principle beyond its limits with an inevitable lack of results.

As homoeopathy has evolved so have the methods of practising, although the principles have remained the same. There are the purists who tend to treat disease by prescribing single remedies which they think best covers the symptoms before them.

This is really the essence of classical homoeopathy as taught by the German doctor, Samuel Hahnemann, the father of this form of medicine.

However, with the vast number of remedies that are now available it becomes increasingly difficult for the practitioner to select the correct remedy in every case. And selecting the wrong remedy means that the patient suffers longer or gives up the treatment.

Those who do not claim to be purists have therefore evolved a system of prescribing several remedies at once which will cover all the symptoms presented by the patient.

Both systems have been adopted by physicians in Europe, but mainly by naturopathic practitioners in Britain.

In my practice I have used a combination of homoeopathic remedies to treat symptoms like hot flushes, depression, weakness, headaches, irregular periods, fluor pruritus vulvae and exhaustion.

CIMICIFUGA

One of the main ingredients of this combination medicine is *Cimicifuga racemosa*, which is a homoeopathic version of the herb Black Cohosh.

In homoeopathy this is indicated as a treatment for the underlying hormonal dysfunction which produces changes in mood and feelings such as restlessness, depression and excitement.

SEPIA

Another of the main ingredients is *Sepia officinalis,* a remedy derived from the fresh ink of the cuttlefish.

Observation shows that this remedy deals with the hormonal effects of the menopause which result in irregular periods, an excessive menstrual flow, feelings of physical tiredness and exhaustion accompanied by a lack of affection for one's partner and family, and hypersensitivity and irritability.

Sepia is the remedy where there is a total disinterest or abhorrence of sexual intercourse. It also gives relief from attacks of perspiration which follow the sudden rushes of heat experienced by some women.

SANGUINARIA

A third ingredient in this homoeopathic mixture is *Sanguinaria canadensis,* known to herbalists as blood root. The homoeopathic potency, or dilution, is prepared from a tincture of the fresh root and is indicated for menopausal headaches, nervous irritability, and feelings of alternating hot and cold.

SULPHURIC

Sulphuric Acid is also indicated, when prepared as a homoeopathic remedy, for hot flushes followed by perspiration, and for vaginal irritation.

LACHESIS

Homoeopaths have long been fascinated by the medicinal values of dilutions of poisonous substances which are used by spiders and snakes to kill their prey.

One such medicine, known as *Lachesis*, is made from the poison produced by one of the deadliest of South American serpents. It is, of course, diluted by homoeopathic pharmacists to a potency that makes it no longer poisonous to humans.

When administered as a remedy during the menopause it seems to help those who complain of feelings of suffocation, oppression and heart weakness – some of the feelings one would get if attacked by such a snake!

It is one of the more important remedies at the menopause as it is also indicated for many of the symptoms, including hot flushes, nervous sensitivity, and general aches and pains. It is reported that *Lachesis* helps to normalise sexual desire by boosting it when it is flagging and reducing it when excessive.

It is also used where there are sudden emotional outbursts and attacks of dizziness.

One effect that snake venom has on its victims is the destruction of the structure of the blood leading to a fatal haemorrhage. In homoeopathy, *Lachesis* is sometimes used to prevent excessive blood loss.

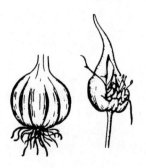

Garlic

Chapter 17

Feed Your Bones

There appears to be a close link between hormones and bones. During the menopause, when oestrogen levels fall, the skeletal system starts to become more brittle because minerals, particularly calcium, are lost from bone.

Eventually, some women may develop the bone disease, osteoporosis, which can be painful and which may put them at a higher risk of suffering a hip fracture should they have a fall.

There is a very strong conviction in medical circles that the menopause will inevitably be followed by osteoporosis unless hormone replacement therapy is instituted on a long-term basis. This is why osteoporosis is considered to be part of what is known as the menopause syndrome.

Some doctors are extremely enthusiastic about oestrogen therapy, believing that this is the best way to prevent hip fractures in elderly women. It is known that oestrogen helps to prevent the breakdown of skeletal tissue unlike thyroxine, the thyroid hormone (see below).

EXERCISE

As a naturopath I have several objections to this line of reasoning. The first is that osteoporosis is a multifactorial disease. There is much more to it than just considering the oestrogens in isolation.

For example, osteoporosis may be caused by lack of exercise. Elderly women who lead active lives are much less likely to develop osteoporosis than those who spend a lot of their time sitting around at home.

This is demonstrated not only by the fact that hospital patients who have to spend many weeks, or months in bed invariably suffer bone loss, but also by studies which show that a moderate exercise regime strengthens bone and protects against osteoporosis.

VITAMIN C

A deficiency of vitamin C is another risk factor for the disease as the vitamin is necessary for the formation of healthy bone tissue. A daily intake of vitamin C is essential as it is rapidly used up by the body. A healthy diet, which includes plenty of fresh fruit and vegetables *all the year round* is highly recommended. If for some digestive reason the diet is low in these items then it would be best to take a natural vitamin C supplement regularly.

VITAMIN D

This vitamin plays a major role in the absorption of calcium from the gastrointestinal tract. Thus a deficiency of vitamin D will lead to a deficiency of calcium. It has been found that bone loss occurs in post-menopausal women whose diet has been low in dairy products and calcium over a period of years.

Conversely, bone loss is halted when calcium and vitamin D supplementation and a proper diet is prescribed. A daily intake of calcium and vitamin D is required. It may be necessary to take supplements for up to four years to achieve proper bone restoration. It should be borne in mind that manufactured vitamin D is toxic in overdose. High doses are not recommended as too much calcium will be absorbed, leading to loss of appetite, muscular weakness, a feeling of sickness and constipation. In addition to dietary sources, vitamin D is made naturally by the body when it is exposed to sunlight. Food sources include fish and fish oils, egg yolk and butterfat. Food sources of calcium include milk, cheese, spinach, beans, broccoli, sweet potato and onion.

Fortunately there has recently been a major advance in the manufacturing process of vitamins and minerals which results in them being more like the nutrients found in food than like isolated chemicals. This means that absorption is greater and the risk of toxicity lower. Much lower doses can therefore be prescribed to achieve the same effect or higher doses can be given without the risk of toxicity. This "food state" method of supplementation is now used by many naturopaths in Britain.

SMOKING

Women smokers tend to experience an earlier meno-pause and a higher incidence of osteoporosis (and other diseases). This is because smoking deprives the body of essential nutrients, including vitamin C. Despite all the health education campaigns, many women continue to smoke with devastating results. If giving up smoking is a problem it can be helped with herbal medicine which reduces the craving for cigarettes by relaxing the system and by making the cigarettes taste unpleasant.

THYROID

Thyroid imbalance becomes more common after the

menopause and should be considered as a possible cause of osteoporosis. If the thyroid becomes over-active the hormones it produces tend to break down body tissue, including bone, leading to the loss of weight.

STEROIDS

The treatment with steroid drugs of a number of conditions, including asthma and skin diseases, has a deleterious effect on bone and is a well known cause of osteoporosis.

The practice of injecting steroids to treat conditions like "frozen shoulder" should be severely restricted, because if it should become necessary to undergo even a minor operation, such as stitching a torn cartilage back into place, it is frequently found by orthopaedic surgeons to be impossible to do because the steroids have "cooked" the tissues with the result that the stitches will not hold in place.

SIGNS AND SYMPTOMS

One of the first symptoms of osteoporosis is back pain, often triggered by an injury or by physical effort such as lifting. It may last for three or four weeks and be wrongly misdiagnosed as sciatica or lumbago. As the disease progresses and more bone is lost the back pain becomes constant due to vertebral fractures.

The back becomes humped and the height shorter. One way of detecting this in most individuals is to measure the distance between the fingertips of one hand to the fingertips of the other when the arms are stretched out sideways. The measurement should be approximately equal to the person's height. In osteoporosis the height becomes significantly less than this measurement, but as some healthy individuals naturally have longer arms any discrepancy between the two measurements may be normal. The measurements usually form only part of a naturopathic investigation.

PREVENTION

Based on the above information the prevention of osteoporosis by naturopathic means would involve a proper health screen to rule out any underlying disease, giving up smoking, taking adequate physical exercise, and following an optimum diet to include fresh fruits and vegetables, fruit juices, and fish and dairy products. Natural food sources of oestrogen (see page 56) should also be used. Where it is seen that a deficiency might exist then supplementation with vitamins and minerals becomes more important.

This seems to be a more sensible approach than the automatic prescription of synthetic oestrogens, which although they may be effective at reducing the risk of hip fractures, have risk factors of their own, including the risk of cancer. However, it is argued that the risk of uterine cancer is minimised by the inclusion of synthetic proges-terone, while any risk of breast cancer is said to be insignificant, and a price worth paying, in view of the reduction in osteoporosis.

Although many family doctors decline to offer HRT as a prevention for osteoporosis, there are constant pressures on them to set up menopausal clinics which could be run by nurses or health visitors. With the population of middle-aged and elderly people set to explode over the next few years it may become more difficult for doctors not to take the easy way out.

In Europe as a whole, calcium supplementation is the most commonly used method of preventing osteoporosis. Even vitamin D supplementation is more popular than oestrogen therapy. French doctors, however, seem to prefer sodium fluoride, despite the fact that it is the least effective of available treatments.

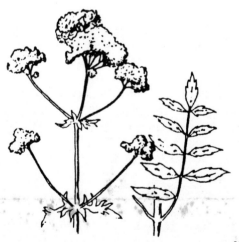

Valerian

Chapter 18

Diet and Supplements

There is no doubt that the kind of diet a woman has followed all her life has an effect on the severity of symptoms at the menopause, and even whether she experiences any symptoms at all.

The fact is that modern diets tend to be deficient in fresh raw foods and in the variety of foods that are used.

I have already pointed out that hormones are part of the complex of substances found in common herbs. In the past herbs were used on a much wider scale as part of everyday food intake – and still are in some parts of the World.

Little scientific research has been done on this, but what has been done shows that the British diet tends to be low in hormonal content, whereas the diets of many people in other parts of the World are rich in oestrogenic substances.

Soya flour, for example, is not consumed in the UK in any great amounts, yet it is a good source of plant oestrogens.

Again, linseed is invariably not the breakfast of choice for UK women, but it contains enough oestrogenic substances for some women to be able to give up HRT. Linseed is available as a breakfast cereal at health stores and adding it to the daily diet is highly recommended.

Because seeds are the plant world's means of reproduction it is logical that this is where one can find a rich supply of plant hormones. Nuts and wheatgerm also come into this category.

I have also explained that the menopause is not just about hormones since symptoms can be alleviated by herbal nervines.

This implies that stress can aggravate the symptoms – and so can diets deficient in nerve vitamins.

I also advise supplementing the diet with the vitamins that are found in seeds, especially vitamin E, which has been found to reduce the severity of hot flushes, pruritus vulvae and the loss of vaginal elasticity.

In addition, vitamin E as part of a healthy diet protects against heart disease.

The diet that I recommend during the menopause excludes devitalised foods and includes plenty of raw vegetable foods, and fruits, compatible with the patient's digestive powers, in order to increase vitamin and mineral intake. Go for wholefoods whenever possible.

So step up your intake of nuts, seeds and wheatgerm and closely related products like wholewheat cereals, and bread, plus soya flour and sprouted seeds and beans. Foods rich in vitamin E, vitamin B and calcium should also be chosen.

Take a "food state" multivitamin and a multimineral supplement every day and, if necessary, supplement with "food state" vitamin E and calcium.

Adequate calcium helps to prevent the onset of osteoporosis.

Chapter 19

Herbal Preparations

Packaged herbal products for the menopause are available from health stores and from other retail outlets, but an individually made up herbal medicine prescribed by a medical herbalist is considered to be superior.

"Teas" made at home from herbs supplied by herbalists may be equally effective.

Most medical herbalists would agree that, where the medicinal properties of a herb are soluble in water, infusions and decoctions are an acceptable way to take them.

They do not agree that home-made or shop bought medicines should be taken on a long-term basis without proper supervision, nor that they should ever be taken for undiagnosed or perhaps serious conditions.

It is also inadvisable to take herbal medicines at the same time as taking medicines from the doctor without appropriate advice as there could be an interaction. This problem is not caused by the herbs, which have been with us for centuries, but by the introduction of compounds and drug molecules unknown in nature.

In making infusions and decoctions care must be taken not to exceed the dosage range of the more potent remedies.

INFUSIONS

Infusions, also known as teas or tisanes, are usually made with the softer parts of the plant, such as the flowers or leaves.

These are chopped finely and about one ounce placed in a jug, or teapot with a close fitting lid. A pint (20 fluid ounces) of boiling water is poured onto the herb and the lid is placed on.

The herb is infused for 10 to 15 minutes, stirring occasionally. When ready the tea is strained off. The usual dosage range is from half to two fluid ounces – that is no more than a small wineglassful – two or three times a day.

If the medicine is to be taken under supervision on a long-term basis half an ounce to one pint of water is usually recommended.

When a combination of herbs is being used to make an infusion the total amount still does not exceed one ounce per pint.

DECOCTIONS

Decoctions are more suitable for the harder parts of the plant, such as the bark, roots and berries. To every ounce of plant material, which is best ground down into a rough powder, or finely chopped 1½ pints (30 fluid ounces) of cold water is poured on and the jug covered. This is then allowed to stand overnight.

The mixture is then brought to the boil and simmered for 20 minutes, or until there is a pint (20 fluid ounces) of liquid left.

The decoction is strained and given in doses of from half to two fluid ounces two or three times a day.

Infusions and decoctions can also be made in a coffee percolator.

TINCTURES

These are used when the medicinal properties of the herb are either destroyed by heat, or not sufficiently soluble in water.

The herb is steeped (macerated) in a mixture (known as the menstruum) of alcohol and cold water – usually a minimum of 20 per cent pure alcohol – for at least two weeks before being pressed out and filtered ready for use.

The tinctures prescribed by medical herbalists are usually made commercially with pure alcohol for which a government licence is necessary. They may also undergo the process of maceration and filtration several times in order to strengthen the tincture and to reduce the final alcohol content to a minimum.

Tinctures can be made with brandy, but this is a rather expensive process. However, the preparation is much stronger than a simple infusion or decoction, the ratio being 1:5 – one ounce of the herb to five fluid ounces of menstruum. Most tinctures need a 25 per cent proportion of alcohol to water. Dosage ranges from 10-40 drops (½ml-2ml), except for the more potent remedies. The advantage of tinctures is that they are more convenient to use and they keep well.

I prefer tinctures made in the ratio of 1:3 – that is one ounce of herb to three fluid ounces of menstruum. On filtration the amount of tincture recovered is made equal to the original amount, i.e. three ounces, by making up the amount with further menstruum, or by re-maceration.

FLUID EXTRACTS

Strong tinctures, or fluid extracts, are made by reducing the final amount of liquid recovered. This is achieved by evaporation of the liquid over a very low heat for several hours using either a water bath, or double saucepan.

An official fluid extract is one that contains the equivalent of one ounce of herb to every fluid ounce of extract (a ratio of 1:1) and contains an adequate amount of alcohol to preserve it.

DOUCHES

Medicinal preparations such as lotions, mouth washes, gargles and douches can be made from infusions. They are filtered after straining off the herb.

INFUSED OILS

Herbs, such as Calendula and Comfrey are steeped in a bland oil, such as olive oil, in a warm place – traditionally in the sun – for at least two weeks so that the medicinal properties are infused into the oil. They are then strained ready for use.

Infused oils are excellent for external use and, therefore, it is perfectly acceptable for the strength to vary. The infusion process can be repeated by adding more herb to the oil and then setting it aside for a further period of time.

A practitioner would use an infused oil of Comfrey, for example, for deep massage and manipulation to the abdomen to improve circulation and to help remove toxic waste from the colon.

This is the oil extracted directly from the plant. They are diluted and used mainly by aromatherapists for simple massage and beauty treatments.

As many essential oils are toxic, even when considerably diluted, they should not be taken internally without expert knowledge.

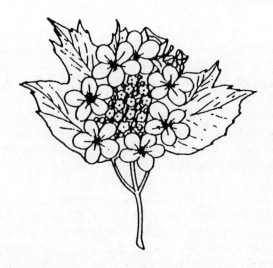

Cramp Bark

Chapter 20

A Herbal Selection

Medical treatment of the menopause did not start with modern hormone replacement therapy. According to medical historians, Egyptian doctors were treating it at least 2000 years ago. Not only did they use medicinal plants, but they also used extracts made from the sex organs of animals.

This might seems strange except that one of the first modern hormone replacement treatments for the menopause, developed in the United States, in the 1940s, was to give women extracts of hormones derived from the urine of horses. These were described – and still are – as natural hormones.

In Britain, the use of medicinal plants has a long history, but today the emphasis is on wholism. The aim of the practitioner is to make up a prescription that takes into account the individual patient and, therefore, each prescription may vary, according to the needs of the particular person being treated.

This section contains a description of botanic remedies frequently prescribed by herbalists to alleviate symptoms associated with the menopause, together with other remedies which have been found to be generally useful.

The correct dosage of some herbs is important and, therefore, they may be available only on private prescription from a medical herbalist.

Agrimony
AGRIMONIA EUPATORIA

Also known as	Church Steeples
Where found	Throughout northern Europe
Appearance	A strong growing herb with green/grey leaves covered with soft hairs. Flowers are small and yellow on long slender spikes.
Part used	Herb
Therapeutic uses	A general tonic which is useful when combined with other indicated remedies in treating simple vaginal discharge and bladder incontinence. The plant is both astringent and diuretic. Used as an infusion the dried leaves are useful in treating simple diarrhoea and general intestinal debility, and to help prevent tissue wasting due to malabsorption.
Prepared as	Tincture, infusion

Alfalfa
MEDICAGO SATIVA

Also known as	Lucerne
Where found	Grows throughout the world.
Appearance	A perennial herb with blue flowers which grows about 18 inches high.
Part used	Leaves

Therapeutic uses   The leaves are rich in vitamins and minerals and are therefore excellent for preventing anaemic conditions. Taken over a period of time, the herb will build up the body. The plant is a good source of natural vitamins C, D, and E, and iron, and also calcium, of which an adequate supply is required by post-menopausal women.

Prepared as   Tincture, infusion, tablets

Avens
GEUM URBANUM

Also known as	Colewort
Where found	Throughout Europe
Appearance	Low-growing herb with yellow flowers
Part used	Herb and root
Therapeutic uses	The plant is astringent, antiseptic, and aromatic, and has a number of uses, including the treatment of leucorrhoea – simple vaginal discharge. An infusion is used as a douche. The decoction applied as a lotion to cuts and wounds stops the bleeding. As a digestive tonic, the infusion can be combined with raspberry and agrimony, or with angelica.
Prepared as	Infusion, decoction, tincture

Bayberry
MYRICA CERIFERA

Also known as	Candle Berry
Where found	United States
Appearance	Shrub up to 8 ft high with shiny leaves and globular berries
Part used	Bark
Therapeutic uses	This remedy improves the blood supply to the uterus and is useful for treating early cases of uterine prolapse. It relieves heavy periods and is also a valuable tonic and cleanser for the whole system. It improves the general circulation and removes catarrh from the stomach. Correct dosage is important.
Prepared as	Powder, fluid extract, tincture, decoction

Beth Root
TRILLIUM PENDULUM

Also known as	Birth Root
Where found	Shady woodlands in the United States
Appearance	A perennial herb producing white flowers which bow down (hence pendulum).
Part used	Root

Therapeutic uses   A uterine astringent which is used to control profuse periods prior to the menopause and bleeding from fibroids. As a douche it is useful in the early stages of uterine prolapse and will control simple vaginal discharges. American Indian women used the remedy during labour to ease childbirth.

Prepared as   Tincture, infusion, powder. Correct dosage is important.

Bistort

POLYGONUM BISTORTA

Also known as	Adderwort
Where found	Europe and northern Britain
Appearance	Low-growing herb chiefly found in ditches and damp places.
Part used	Root
Therapeutic uses	A powerful astringent due to its high content of tannin. It has a general tonic action, but is mainly used as an anti-diarrhoeal. It is also used in incontinence and to check leucorrhoea. As a gargle, it eases sore throats.
Prepared as	Tincture, fluid extract, decoction

Black Cohosh
CIMICIFUGA RACEMOSA

Also known as	Squaw Root
Where found	United States and Canada
Appearance	A tall herbaceous plant with white feathery flowers
Part used	Rhizome
Therapeutic uses	Mainly known as a "woman's remedy" – it improves the menstrual flow. It is also used as a general blood purifier and nervine tonic, with antispasmodic, anti-flatuent and sedative properties. It is used in small doses as large doses may cause nausea and vomiting. Contraindicated in pregnancy.
Prepared as	Infusion, decoction, syrup, tincture

Bladderwrack
FUCUS VESICULOSIS

Also known as	Seawrack or Kelp
Where found	Around the coasts of Britain
Appearance	A large trailing seaweed, dark green in colour
Part used	Dried plant
Therapeutic uses	Stimulates the thyroid gland, most likely because of its iodine content. Its reputation as a

slimming agent is probably also due to its stimulant effect on this gland.

Prepared as   Tincture, decoction

Borage
BORAGO OFFICINALIS

Also known as	Burrage
Where found	Throughout Europe
Appearance	A bold, erect herb of strong growth. Small blue flowers.
Part used	Leaves, seeds
Therapeutic uses	A remedy for cyclical headaches and migraine. It is a stimulating tonic, which is reputed to aid the adrenal glands – the glands of stress. It is also demulcent and diuretic. The oil extracted from the seeds is similar to evening primrose oil in that it contains gamma-linolenic acid (GLA), which has been found useful in treating several conditions, including premenstrual tension, painful breasts and other menstrual upsets. The amount of GLA in borage oil, however, is greater than that found in evening primrose oil and may become more popular in the future.
Prepared as	Infusion, oil (from seeds)

Buchu
BAROSMA BETULINA

Also known as	Bookoo
Where found	Western coast of South Africa
Appearance	Small procumbent herb growing in dry places.
Part used	Leaves
Therapeutic uses	A medicine for the urinary tract and bladder. It is an important item in the modern herbalist's dispensary, as it is a good remedy for cystitis. It has a mild, stimulating diuretic action and is also antiseptic. The infusion and tincture were once official medicines listed in the British Pharmacopoeia. It is often combined with more potent remedies depending on the condition being treated.
Prepared as	Infusion, tincture

Burdock
ARCTIUM LAPPA

Also known as	Beggar's Buttons
Where found	Britain and Europe
Appearance	Strong growing plant with large leaves.
Part used	Roots, seeds and leaves

Therapeutic uses	One of the best blood purifiers and dermatological agents. It is used extensively in skin conditions, often in combination with Sarsaparilla and Yellow Dock. A lesser known use is its ability to improve the tone of vaginal tissue. The tincture is taken internally and a compress soaked in a decoction is applied externally.
Prepared as	Tincture, decoction, infusion

Cardamom
ELETTARIA CARDAMOMUM

Also known as	Malabar Cardamom
Where found	Ceylon and India
Appearance	Forest plant with large smooth, dark green leaves and small yellowish flowers
Part used	Fruits, seeds and oil
Therapeutic uses	An aromatic herb mainly used in the treatment of flatulence and to aid digestion. Small amounts are added to other medicines to improve their palatability. Cardamom also has a reputation as a sexual tonic and is incorporated into medicines for this purpose.
Prepared as	Powder, liquid extract, tincture

Chamomile, Wild
MATRICARIA CHAMOMILLA

Also known as	German Chamomile
Where found	Corn fields in Europe
Appearance	Herb with small cushion-like flowers in profusion
Part used	Flowers
Therapeutic uses	An excellent nerve sedative and a valuable gastro-intestinal tonic. It is used for headaches and migraine, especially when due to food intolerance. Chamomile also has carminative and antispasmodic properties. It reduces flatulence and abdominal distension and eases colicky pains and spasms in the colon. Continual daily use is indicated where there is inflammation.
Prepared as	Infusion, tincture

Chamomile, Common
ANTHEMIS NOBILIS

Also known as	Belgian Chamomile
Where found	A favourite garden herb, abundant in France and Belgium, but widely cultivated.
Appearance	A herb resembling a large daisy with white flowers and yellow centres.

Part used	Flowers and herb
Therapeutic uses	Widely prescribed for nervous and hysterical conditions. It is an antispasmodic indicated in stomach and intestinal disorders. Very useful in heartburn, simple indigestion, flatulence, colic, and debilitated states of the colon.
Prepared as	Infusion (chamomile tea), fluid extract, tincture

Cinnamon
CINNAMOMUM ZEYLANICUM

Where found	A native plant of Ceylon
Appearance	A tree growing up to 30ft high in sandy soils
Part used	Bark
Therapeutic uses	A pleasantly aromatic herb with carminative, antiseptic, and astringent properties. An effective remedy for vomiting and nausea, and will give relief in flatulence and diarrhoea.
Prepared as	Oil, medicinal water, tincture, powder

Cramp Bark
VIBURNUM OPULUS

Also known as	Snowball tree, Guelder rose

Where found	Europe and the United States
Appearance	Strong-growing bush with white ball-shaped flowers
Part used	Bark
Therapeutic uses	Cramp bark, as its name suggests, is an antispasmodic. It is also an excellent nervine and has been used to treat spasms and convulsions.
Prepared as	Decoction and tincture

Cranesbill
GERANIUM MACULATUM

Also known as	Wild Geranium or Storksbill
Where found	United States
Appearance	Shrubby small herb with blue flowers. The seed pod resembles a crane's bill.
Part used	Herb and root
Therapeutic uses	An astringent used in the treatment of menstrual flooding. An infusion of the herb is made with equal parts of Cranesbill and Beth Root and used as a douche. On its own Cranesbill is healing to the stomach and intestines, particularly if the bowels are loose and there is catarrhal discharge and bleeding. It makes a useful treatment for piles. Avoid large doses internally.

Prepared as	Infusion (of herb), decoction (of root), powder, tincture

Echinacea
ECHINACEA ANGUSTIFOLIA

Also known as	Cone Flower
Where found	American prairies
Appearance	Herb of medium height
Part used	Rhizome
Therapeutic uses	Natural antibiotic, antiseptic and alterative. It increases the body's resistance to infection. Helps to clear the blood of toxic material. Improves appetite and digestion. Used in ulcerative conditions of the stomach and duodenum to keep the tissues clean. Can be combined with small amount of Goldenseal.
Prepared as	Decoction and tincture. Correct dosage is important.

Garlic
ALLIUM SATIVUM

Where found	Universally cultivated
Appearance	Similar to a shallot
Part used	Bulb

Therapeutic uses	Protects the heart by reducing blood cholesterol. It is a powerful antiseptic.
Prepared as	Powder, oil (in capsules), juice, tablets and tincture

Gentian
GENTIANA LUTEA

Also known as	Yellow gentian
Where found	Alpine plant in Europe
Appearance	A hardy herbaceous perennial bearing clusters of large orange-yellow flowers.
Part used	Root
Therapeutic uses	One of the finest tonics, but intensely bitter even when greatly diluted. It improves the menstrual flow, stimulates appetite and aids digestion. Often prescribed when there is a general debility and jaundice. A useful remedy for dyspepsia. It is better to combine small doses of the medicine with an aromatic herb such as Cardamom to help camouflage the bitter taste.
Prepared as	Tincture and powder (use a quarter of a teaspoonful infused in a cupful of boiling water and sweetened with honey).

Ginger
ZINGIBER OFFICINALE

Where found	West Indies and China
Appearance	About one metre high with glossy aromatic leaves
Part used	Rhizome
Therapeutic uses	An excellent remedy for indigestion. Ginger is mainly used in small doses as a carminative – it reduces flatulence and distension and eases painful intestinal spasms. It also reduces fermentation in the bowel.
Prepared as	Powder, syrup, tablets and tincture

Goldenseal
HYDRASTIS CANADENSIS

Also known as	Yellow Root
Where found	Cultivated in North America
Appearance	Tall-growing herb with disagreeable odour
Part used	Rhizome
Therapeutic uses	A most important medicinal herb. It is particularly soothing to the epithelium – the skin surface both outside and inside the body, including mouth, throat, stomach, intestinal lining, uterus and

vagina. It is antiseptic, antifungal, laxative and purifies the blood. It is used with other indicated remedies for vaginitis and inflammation of the cervix. As a tonic it helps those with irritable and inflammatory conditons of the stomach and colon. It is indicated in most digestive disorders. Small doses only are used. It is contraindicated in pregnancy.

Prepared as   Tincture, decoction, powder

Hops
HUMULUS LUPULUS

Where found	Cultivated in most parts of the world
Appearance	A climbing vine
Part used	Strobile
Therapeutic uses	A nervine tonic and sedative with oestrogenic action. Mainly used in combination with other remedies for treatment of the menopause, particularly where there is restlessness. It allays pain and promotes restful sleep. Correct dosage is important.
Prepared as	Tincture, infusion

Lady's Slipper
CYPRIPEDIUM PUBESCENS

Also known as	Nerve Root
Where found	Europe and the United States
Appearance	A delicate wild orchid at present in short supply and, therefore, highly expensive. Attempts to grow it commercially for medicinal use have not been very successful.
Part used	Rhizome
Therapeutic uses	A most effective nervine used to allay disorders of a nervous origin, including emotional tension. It helps to induce natural sleep. It is also antispasmodic and relaxing.
Prepared as	Powder, decoction, fluid extract and tincture

Lemon Balm
MELISSA OFFICINALIS

Also known as	Sweet Balm
Where found	A common garden herb
Appearance	It belongs to the nettle family to which it bears some resemblance. The leaves emit a strong lemon smell when rubbed or crushed.
Part used	Leaves, whole herb

Therapeutic uses	Carminative. A useful and safe remedy for the stomach. It relieves flatulence and gastric upsets. It has antifungal properties and is also indicated in fevers. It will induce sweating. An infusion of the leaves (one ounce to one pint of boiling water) can be drunk as required.
Prepared as	Infusion

Pulsatilla
ANEMONE PULSATILLA

Also known as	Wind Flower
Where found	Britain and Europe
Part used	Leaves
Therapeutic uses	Sedative, nervine, antispasmodic. Helpful for women with menstrual and menopausal problems and also for headaches associated with tension. Also indicated for insomnia and skin eruptions. Small doses only to be used.
Prepared as	Tincture (to be taken under medical supervision).

Raspberry
RUBUS IDAEUS

Where found	Common in gardens in most temperate climates

Appearance	A bush producing edible fruit
Part used	Leaves
Therapeutic uses	Astringent and stimulant. Its hormonal-like action explains its traditional use for easier and speedier labour in childbirth. As a uterine relaxant it gives relief to those who suffer painful periods. It is mild in action and soothing to the mucous lining of the stomach and intestinal tract. Contraindicated in early pregnancy.
Prepared as	Tincture, infusion (which may be used as a douche)

Red Sage
SALVIA OFFICINALIS

Also known as	Garden Sage
Where found	Commonly cultivated as a culinary herb in Europe and the United States.
Appearance	A herb growing to about 12cm with purplish flowers
Part used	Leaves
Therapeutic uses	Traditionally a fertility herb, it has an oestrogenic action. It has been used in menstrual disorders, including painful periods, absence of periods, and simple vaginal discharge. It also helps prevent excessive perspiration and is a useful remedy during the

menopause. Although widely available as a culinary herb, it is recommended only for short-term use as a medicine. It should not be taken during pregnancy.

Prepared as   Infusion and tincture

Rosemary
ROSMARINUS OFFICINALIS

Where found	A well known garden herb
Appearance	A shrubby herb with evergreen spiky leaves and small pale blue flowers
Part used	Leaves
Therapeutic uses	Rosemary is an effective treatment to increase the menstrual flow, but it should not be used in pregnancy. An infusion of a few leaves to a cup of boiling water (infuse for a few minutes only) will ease headaches due to stomach upsets. It also eases flatulence and is antifungal.
Prepared as	Tincture, infusion

Valerian
VALERIAN OFFICINALIS

Also known as	All Heal
Where found	Near streams, rivers and ditches in Britain

Appearance	Grows to about a metre in height with pinkish white flowers
Part used	Rhizome
Therapeutic uses	A nervine, sedative and antispasmodic which is frequently used in the menopause. Excellent for relieving nervous tension and debility and for promoting sleep. It also helps to improve the menstrual flow. Correct dosage is important.
Prepared as	Decoction, fluid extract and tincture

Vervain
VERBENA OFFICINALIS

Also known as	Herb of Grace
Where found	By roadsides and in meadows in Britain
Appearance	A perennial trailing herb bearing small pale-lilac flowers
Part used	Leaves
Therapeutic uses	An excellent nervine, helping to lift depression and ease tension. It also improves the menstrual flow and eases painful menstrual periods.
Prepared as	Infusion and tincture

Wild Yam
DIOSCOREA VILLOSA

Also known as	Colic Root
Where found	Tropical countries, United States and Canada
Appearance	A perennial climbing plant.
Part used	Root
Therapeutic uses	An antispasmodic which relieves uterine pain. Also useful in neuralgia. It contains a hormone-like compound which has been used in the manufacture of the contraceptive pill. *Caution: large doses may induce vomiting.*
Prepared as	Decoction, fluid extract and tincture. Note: dried root quickly loses its therapeutic potency.

Wood Betony
BETONICA OFFICINALIS

Also known as	Bishopswort
Where found	Woodland in Europe
Appearance	A broad-leaved plant with spikes of red flowers spotted white
Part used	Leaves, or whole herb
Therapeutic uses	A general tonic particularly useful in conditions where both nerves and stomach are involved, such as stomach pain and headaches due

to digestive upsets. Helps alleviate dyspepsia.

Prepared as   Decoction, infusion and tincture

Yarrow
ACHILLEA MILLEFOLIUM

Also known as	Nosebleed, Milfoil, Thousand-Leaf
Where found	Roadsides, meadows and waste ground in Britain
Appearance	An upright plant growing to about 61cm with leaves divided into a multitude of parts, hence the name thousand-leaf. The flowers are white or pink with yellowish centres.
Part used	Herb
Therapeutic uses	An astringent which helps to correct excessively heavy periods, treat simple vaginal discharge and tone up vaginal tissue. The tincture is usually used in combination with other remedies. The hot infusion induces sweating making it an excellent remedy in colds, flu and catarrh: combine with peppermint.
Prepared as	Cold infusion, hot infusion (for colds), tincture

Chapter 21

Seeking Professional Help

Although this book is aimed at giving those with menopausal problems information and guidance on the herbal and naturopathic approach to treatment, it cannot be stressed too much that quicker results can often be achieved by consulting a fully qualified herbal or naturopathic practitioner.

When treatment is being conducted by a medical herbalist the functioning of the whole body will be taken into account and, therefore, the prescription will vary from one individual to another.

Patients are seen by appointment and in confidence in the practitioner's consulting rooms. Herbal practitioners qualified with the National Institute of Medical Herbalists, can be recognised by the initials MNIMH or FNIMH after their names.

They are trained to deal with a wide range of medical problems, although some practitioners may specialise in certain medical areas.

Naturopaths trained at the British College of Naturopathy and Osteopathy in London and admitted to the Register of Naturopaths have the letters ND MRN after their names.

They are specialists in the non-drug treatment of a wide variety of conditions, although many naturopaths are also qualified osteopaths and tend to specialise in musculo-skeletal problems.

The National Institute of Medical Herbalists, founded in 1864, is the oldest established body of practising medical herbalists in the world. Members can be found in most towns in the UK. The easiest way to find out if there is one near you is to look under 'Herbalists' in Yellow Pages, Thomson's, or other local directory.

The aim of both naturopathy and herbal medicine is not just to relieve symptoms but to offer the sufferer an increased level of general health. Practitioners take an holistic approach to their patients, an approach that is being followed more and more by other primary health care practitioners.

They will, therefore, take into account not only the physical symptoms of the menopause but also any mental stress or emotional problems which may be relevant.

FURTHER READING

Other books in this series include:

Skin Problems
Arthritis and Rheumatism
Stress and Tension
Sexual Problems
Irritable Bowel Syndrome
Hiatus Hernia
Asthma

Glossary of Common Medical Terms

Very often when reading, or on having a medical consultation, words are used which may not be familiar. This short list will help to make some of the more common ones a little clearer.

Alterative   A medicine that beneficially alters the process of nutrition and restores the normal function of an organ or bodily system. In herbal medicine it usually refers to a remedy that purifies the blood by improving the function of the organs, such as liver and kidneys, which are involved in this process.

Amenorrhoea   Absence of menstrual periods during the years when they should normally be present.

Analgesic   A medicine that blocks or relieves pain.

Anodyne   A medicine that alleviates pain – physical or mental.

Anthelmintic   A medicine that is used to rid the body of intestinal worms.

Antiphlogistic   A medicine, or agent, which reduces inflammation or fever.

Antipyretic A medicine, or method, used to lower the body temperature to normal. In naturopathic medicine, cold baths, and spongeing or application of ice packs are used to combat fever.

Antiseptic A medicine, or other substance, that prevents putrefaction.

Antispasmodic A remedy that prevents or relieves colic or spasms. Among the most potent antispasmodics derived from plants are belladonna and opium. Naturopathic antispasm is achieved with the application of hot compresses and fomentations.

Aperient A remedy that produces a natural movement of the bowels.

Aphrodisiac A substance that is reputed to produce sexual desire and stimulate the sexual organs.

Astringent Binding or contracting tissues.

Cardiac Relating to the heart, either a medicine, or disease, that alters heart function.

Carminative A medicine that eases griping pains and flatulence in the bowel.

Cathartic A strong laxative, or purgative, producing evacuation of the bowels.

Climacteric The whole transition period during which a woman's fertility declines and ceases and other bodily changes take place which eventually lead to senescence.

Corrective	Correcting or counteracting the harmful and restoring to a healthy state.
Debility	Feebleness of health; run down.
Degenerative	A disease that results in destruction or disintegration of tissue.
Demulcent	A soothing medicine, mostly applied to those that act on the gastrointestinal canal.
Deobstruent	Removing obstructions and opening the ducts and other natural passages of the body.
Diaphoretic	A substance that induces perspiration.
Diuretic	A substance that increases the flow of urine.
Dysmenorrhoea	Excessive pain during menstruation
Dyspnoea	Breathlessness
Emetic	Any substance that causes vomiting.
Emmenagogue	A remedy that brings on the menstrual period.
Emollient	A medicine that softens, soothes and lubricates skin and internal tissues.
Haematemesis	Vomiting of blood
Haemoptysis	Coughing up of blood
Haemostatic	A substance that checks bleeding and aids clotting of the blood.
Insecticide	Any substance fatal to insects.
Laxative	A substance that induces gentle, and easy bowel movement.

Leucorrhoea	A mucous discharge from the female genital organs, previously known as "the whites".
Menorrhagia	Excessive flow of menstrual blood.
Menopause	The final menstrual period.
Metrorrhagia	Irregular bleeding from the uterus not associated with menstruation.
Myalgia	Muscular pain; muscular rheumatism.
Narcotic	A drug that produces drowsiness, sleep, stupor and insensibility.
Nephritic	Relating to the kidneys.
Nervine	A remedy that relieves a nerve disorder and restores the nervous system to its normal state.
Oxytocic	A drug that causes contractions of the uterus and hastens childbirth.
Parturient	A remedy used during childbirth.
Purgative	A medicine taken to evacuate the bowels, but one that is much stronger than a laxative or aperient.
Resolvent	A drug, application, or other substance that reduces swellings and tumours.
Rubefacient	A treatment that produces redness, inflammation and blisters of the skin; a counter-irritant (rubefy = make red).
Sedative	A remedy soothing to the nervous system; a tranquilliser.
Soporific	Promoting sleep.
Stimulant	A remedy that produces a rapid

increase in vital energy of part or of the whole body.

Stomachic
Relating to the stomach; a remedy that aids the normal function of the stomach, promoting proper digestion and appetite.

Stricture
The narrowing of any of the natural passages of the body, such as the urethra, the bowel or the gullet.

Styptic
A substance that checks bleeding.

Sudorific
A remedy that produces heavy perspiration.

Tonic
A medicine that invigorates or tones up a part or the whole of the body and promotes wellbeing.

Vermifuge
A medicine that expels worms from the body.

Vulnerary
An ointment or treatment that promotes the healing of wounds.

The Author

David Potterton is one of a few practitioners in Britain who are qualified in both herbal and naturopathic medicine. He has practices in Reading and Wokingham, Berkshire.

A member of the National Institute of Medical Herbalists (NIMH) and of the British Naturopathic Association (BNA), he is also member of the General Council and Register of Naturopaths.

Mr Potterton has been a member of the McCarrison Society – a medical organisation devoted to the study of health and nutrition – for several years.

He was also a member of the Royal Society of Medicine for many years and a member of the Vegetarian Society's research committee.

Mr Potterton has been tutor for the NIMH, and has conducted a series of further education lecture courses on herbal medicine. He also lectures frequently to local organisations and health workers in the Thames Valley.

As a writer, Mr Potterton has contributed to all the major health magazines in the UK, including *"Here's Health"* and *"Healthy Living"*, and was the English editor of *"Bestways"*, the American health magazine, as well as being a contributor to the *"US Quarterly Journal of Health"*.

He was medical editor of the family doctor newspaper *"Doctor"* for many years, and co-editor of the *"British Journal of Phytotherapy"*, a professional journal for herbal practitioners and naturopathic physicians both in the UK and abroad.

He is the editor of several books published by Foulsham, including *"Culpeper's Colour Herbal"* and *"Medicinal Plants"*.

He has also revised and edited a number of Foulsham books on herbal medicine in this series, including *"Arthritis and Rheumatism"*, *"Skin Problems"*, *"Stress and Tension"* and *"Sexual Problems"*. He is also the author of three other books in this series, *"Irritable Bowel Syndrome"*, *"Asthma"* and *"Hiatus Hernia"*.

Your Story

If you have benefited from the use of herbal medicines during the menopause, either from home use or from those prescribed by professional medical herbalists or naturopaths, you are invited to send details to the author of this series of books, c/o the publishers, W. Foulsham & Co. Ltd, The Publishing House, Bennetts Close, Cippenham, Berkshire SL1 5AP.